CONTENTS

In this book, I will share
5 wrong mindsets and 5
solutions in achieving a
consistent healthy lifestyle
through my experiences and
the clients I have trained
over the years. Mindset
is the foundation to your
success and failures not only
in your health but in the
rest of your life as well.

ABOUT THE AUTHOR

My name is John Te, I have been a personal trainer since 2013, started my career in a commercial gym. Where I was a fitness manager at three different locations for three out of the four years I worked there. I left there 2017 to venture out on my own but also took a job as a personal trainer for Johnson and Johnson for one year until I decided the direction I wanted to go in. I officially started Execution Fitness March 2018.

My story will be broken into two parts. The person before fitness and the current person helping you today. I was always a skinny kid growing up, I didn't think much of it, most kids around me were skinny at that age. As years went on kids got bigger and taller, at least that's how it's supposed to go. I got taller but not bigger when I started high school is when I noticed how skinny I was compared to the other kids, which made me insecure. I lacked confidence and self-esteem, during that time of my life, I cared too much of what my peers thought of me and felt I was someone whom other kids didn't want to be around because of how skinny I was, at least that's what I fabricated internally. I wasn't actually bullied about being skinny, the only thing I remember is a girl telling me she wouldn't go out with me because I was skinny but that's the only relevant circumstance I remember. In my mind, though I wasn't good enough until I was of "normal weight". This insecurity actually started at home, my parents would get mad at me for being so thin and yell at me for not eating, it's not that I didn't want to eat, I just didn't like what my parents cooked and I find this is the case for my clients who are 16 years of age and below but that's for a later time. I played baseball growing and had an uncle that told me I didn't swing that bat the bat swung me, this didn't bother me that much at the time but the seed was planted. My parents made it more clear how skinny I was compared to the other kids in my age group as high school went on. I was roughly 110 pounds my senior year of high school, I'm about five foot, six. By this time that seed of insecurity blossomed, I didn't participate in any of my school activities or functions through my years in high school, even prom. Looking back on this time of my life I wasn't in a good mental state. I didn't really know it but I was suppressing my feelings about myself, about my parents, about why me? Why can't I just be normal and not skinny? I'm sure some of you have felt like this in life, whether being skinny or big we all have our insecurities. Finishing up my story, I was starting college and now that I would be living at school, I can eat whatever I wanted to eat, no more being skinny! I decided to do something about it, I started to educate myself, reading fitness article after fitness article, watching fitness video after fitness video. I was like many of you, overwhelmed by the amount of information, so I tried a couple of things but like most people I was bouncing around from one exercise program and diet to another. I saw results, two and a half months in I put on 20 pounds which put me around 130 pounds. I was still confused about all I read and watched but something was working I wasn't as skinny anymore, had a little muscle definition, my confidence and self-esteem grew as well. The rest of college I saw how my body transformed from a skinny kid into someone with more confidence because of exercise.

PART 2:

Towards the end of my college career, I was watching the Biggest Loser where I saw a lot of broken people and I saw what the trainers did for them mentally and physically. I knew what it felt like, not to that extreme but I knew how mentally challenging it was as well as physically. As I kept watching the show it became clearer to me that achieving a healthy lifestyle was more mental than physical, exactly what I went through. It wasn't that they couldn't run or do any of the exercises it was their mindset holding them back, sometimes deeper insecurities that was suppressed, that needed to be addressed more so than the physical body. I've now been a trainer since 2013, I've worked at your typical gym as a trainer and a fitness manager for 4 years, then worked at Johnson and Johnson's headquarters training their corporate employees for 1 year. I started Execution Fitness because I wanted to take what I learned personally and professionally and help more people like yourself. Becoming and staying healthy is not complicated, I aim to simplify that process so you can live a long healthy life.

ExecutionFitness.com

THOUGHT 1: YOU DON'T BELIEVE YOU CAN ACHIEVE!

◆ ◆ ◆

Do you believe you can achieve your goals?

There are a limitless amount of FREE workout and nutrition programs out in the world so why do people still struggle with their health? It does not matter whether you are on the keto diet, south beach diet, intermittent fasting, going to kickboxing, following a 30-day program or if you are working with a personal trainer. Nothing, I repeat NOTHING will work unless YOU BELIEVE you can achieve your goals!

This is where in the countless consultations I have done over the years I have seen a lack of confidence when I go over people's goals. "I can't work out on my own.", "I don't know if I can lose 20lbs, let's start with 5lbs.", "Doctor says I'll always have this pain.", "I'll never be able to get off this medication." Body language and defeated tone when discussing their goals, it was like there was no way they could achieve the goals and just said them because I asked for their goals. They did not believe they could achieve them! Failure has already been declared before starting! How many of you do this? If you wonder why you have not progressed in your fitness goals and maybe your life goals as well are because of this wrong mindset. This thinking stems from past failures that you may have experienced or by hearing or seeing other people fail around you. Maybe you did try a workout and nutrition program and it did not work for you, that does not dictate that any program you try after that will not work. You have to keep trying, believing that this time around is when you will reach your goals. Letting past failures prevent you from trying is like not driving again after getting into an accident. Let me ask you this: Does working out and eating right get you closer or further away from your goals? I'm sure that the answer would be obvious but why when a program does not work out we quit entirely? Maybe your answer is, "I don't want to be doing something that's not working". I can empathize and sympathize with that but reverting to doing nothing is not the answer. Instead change your mindset to, "I'm determined to reach my goal.", "Let me find something that works for me and ask for help." and "Let me continue to do what I know to do until I find a plan that works for me." The latter is crucial, keep exercising, keep eating right until you find the program that works for you. We overcomplicate health, you know the difference between pizza and a salad, you know you should be moving more. Start creating good habits then bad habits will fall away naturally and believe you can achieve and say positive things! Do not sit around with your friends and complain about your health issues, wearing them as if they are some sort of badge in your life, "My back pain.", "My knee pain.", "My fat stomach." It is ok to be frustrated but discuss solutions not just about what is going wrong. Shift to positive conversations, "I'm not losing weight right now but I'll get some help.", "I'll get off this blood pressure medication.", "I'll lose 50lbs, I know I can." Where the mind goes that body follows. Now just like your body, your mindset also takes time to change but the more you say positive things, think positive thoughts and surround yourself with positive people, the closer your actions will reflect your thoughts and words. Nothing is accomplished by staying negative, it keeps you stuck!

A healthier you starts and ends here if you still do not believe you can achieve your goals, nothing you read or do after this will matter. Re-read this first step until it really sinks in. Mindset is the foundation for maintaining a sustainable, healthy lifestyle.

THOUGHT 2: YOU DON'T KNOW WHY...

◆ ◆ ◆

Why do you want to become healthy?

I often get the question, "How do you stay motivated?" The real question is Why? Why do I workout 6-7 days a week and eat healthy most of the week? And been doing so since 2008. In that time span, my WHY has evolved and to achieve a healthy lifestyle will require your WHY to evolve as well. I was a skinny kid, heading into my freshman year of college I was roughly 110 pounds. At that time my goals were to get bigger without getting a belly. Why? I was insecure and wanted to get girls and just didn't want to be skinny anymore! The problem? Somedays I cared about my why and some days I didn't so the results were sporadic. Some days I went to the gym, some days I didn't, some days I ate healthily and some days I didn't. Sound like most of you? Your body reflects what you are most consistent with and healthy habits occur when your why is in focus, every day not some days. How has my why changed since then? Since I've been a trainer in 2013 I have done countless consultations, I have seen every type of person, from young to old and all types of health issues. I've seen what happens when you do not take care of yourself, broken relationships, marriages, medication after medication being taken on a daily basis, mentally broken, people who have cried because of their health issues. I have seen and heard too much not to take care of myself and this is my message to you, do not wait until you have a life-altering diagnosis before you start taking care of yourself. Healthy habits are the best insurance plan. This is why your WHY matters! I have seen and heard about people who make terrific progress, lose 100lbs, get off medications but revert back to old ways once they reach their ultimate goal or have made significant progress towards it. For example, at my commercial gym, we had 3-month contracts for personal training. I would sometimes see clients make great progress over the 3 months only to see them inconsistent or never come back to the gym after their contract was finished! Partly this was on me as a trainer not keeping up with my former clients, I was young and have grown since then but part of it also was they lost focus on their why. I'm sure none of you reading this want to lose weight or make progress in your health only for a temporary period. This is the reason it is very crucial to remain focused on your why not your goals. Your goals will be achieved when you are focused on your why.

You have to have a deep reason why you want to improve your health, the reason has to impact you in a profound way. Just like my first why in college to my why now, big difference and the latter impacts me in such a profound way and that what keeps me going. In my career, the people who achieved and maintained a healthy lifestyle could tell me with passion why they are doing what they are doing. The key word there is "passion", you have to care about your why you have to prioritize your why especially on the days where you do not "feel" like it. I'll be addressing your "feelings" later.

"I want to become healthy." is too general, I'm sure everyone reading this wants to be healthy in some way shape or form. Let's get specific with it, " I want to become healthy for my kids so I can be active with them and watch them grow up and get married and see my grandkids." Now, which is more impactful to you? What resonates to other people when they ask you why you workout five days a week and eat healthy as you do? Now write it down, your goals become real when you can see it, knowing you wrote it and no one forced you. Create a list then go over your reasons and be honest with yourself, are your goals superficial or are they meaningful? For example, if you wrote down, "I want to look better and feel better." Ask yourself why do I want to look better and feel better? Get to the root, it will most likely be painful, there might be some unresolved issues in your past that is buried inside you. This is poison, in order to move forward, you have to accept yourself where you are, knowing you are making a change for the better. Just like your physical body takes time to change so does your mindset. Change does not happen overnight and it is a painful process but I guarantee you do not want to stay where you are or why else are you reading this? Where you are right now, even though it is not where you want to be, is because you have accepted your current state as normal and have become comfortable with the habits that have come along with it. You know you need to make a change but that requires being uncomfortable, in order to push through is the reasons WHY you want to make a change! Put your goals somewhere where you can see it every day, that becomes a promise to yourself, believe you can achieve them and that starts to shift your mindset.

THOUGHT 3: YOU LET FEELINGS RULE YOU

◆ ◆ ◆

How do you feel?

We are a society run by our feelings. "I don't feel good.", "I feel tired.", "I'm not in the mood to eat healthy." It usually starts out with, "I feel..." then something negative. Sound like you? Goes back to the end of step 1: MINDSET. Negativity does not progress you closer towards your goal. For example, I've had a long day at work and I know I should go to the gym but I really don't "feel" like it. I've been there, I still have those feelings, you don't need motivation, you need discipline. It goes back to my question in step 1: Does working out and eating right get you closer or further away from your goals? I didn't ask how you felt about it. You know you should go but feelings prevent you from going then snowballs into the rest of the week and before you know it you skipped a whole week and ate terribly. Motivation gets you started but discipline is what separates the successful people. One of the many meanings of discipline is self-control. The meaning of self-control: restraint exercised over one's own impulses, emotions, or desires. Emotion is a synonym for feelings! You have to restrain your emotions/feelings on a daily basis, that means sticking with your workout and nutrition program no matter the circumstances inward or outward. I can hear it now, "It's too hard!" This is where your "Why" gets tested. At this moment where you feel it's too hard for you, does your why mean anything to you? If you have to think about it, it is not important enough to you. Every day we run on a schedule and that schedule is based on importance, work, kids, meetings, grocery shopping, etc. Exercise and eating healthy, in my experiences are the first ones to go when life gets "busy". That means your why does not mean enough to you for you to prioritize it. If this is you re-read step 2. Feelings are fickle, just because you feel a certain way doesn't mean it is the truth. Do you know why you are always tired? It could be you don't get enough sleep but if you do it is because you keep telling yourself, you're tired! No one talks to you more than yourself. Your thoughts are conversations with yourself. Think about what you are thinking about. Back to step 1 and nega-tivity, are your thoughts perpetually negative? If yes, you are more likely to cave into those nega-tive emotions. How do we change this? Talk back to yourself and say positive things, you control your thoughts, you don't have to think about anything that pops into your head, change the channel to something positive. Meditate on your why and the reasons behind it, imagine how great your life will be when your goals are achieved. Positivity always wins.

THOUGHT 4: I FAILED!

◆ ◆ ◆

What do you do when you're following a program and it's not working?

Realize success is not linear, you are human and therefore you are not perfect, you will have days where you completely fail. If you did not workout and ate poorly, the program is not ruined. Often the mindset is, "I'll start back up Monday." or you'll let it snowball into more bad decisions. Change the mindset to start making the next healthy choice as soon as possible. If you ate a bad lunch, have a good dinner. If you missed your morning workout, see if you have some time later in the day. Do not let negative feelings and thoughts flood your mind when you fail, failure is part of the process. Allow yourself to fail and when you accept that it is part of your journey, refocus on your why, then the easier it will be to get back on track. Becoming healthy is not about depriving yourself, I preach this to my clients, enjoy your life and do not feel guilty when you eat poorly or miss a workout. Always keep in mind your body reflects what you are more CONSISTENT with. For example, if you eat 3 meals a day that's 21 meals in a week if you ate poorly 3 of those meals, that's 14% of your total meals. Now I am not saying you are allowed 3 bad meals especially if you are not disciplined yet but what I am saying is 3 bad meals amongst 18 good meals won't impede your progress. Focus on being consistent not on being perfect. If you focus on being perfect you don't allow yourself to fail and when you inevitably do fail, it demoralizes you. Whereas if you focus on being consistent you can immediately identify the problem then reverse your habits back to what you need to be doing.

THOUGHT 5: RESULTS ARE TAKING TOO LONG!

◆ ◆ ◆

<u>Sic Parvis Magna:</u>
"Greatness from small beginnings."

Are you patient with yourself?

Achieving your goals is a step by step process and those steps are small, there is no instant change overnight, physically or mentally. You must accept that you are where you are because of the decisions YOU have made and blame no one else. Accept responsibility for where you are, now I realize some of you have been dealt a bad hand but the great news is YOU have the power to change the narrative on your life. If you do not like where you are, make that DECISION that you will make every effort to change no matter how hard the road gets. For me, it was a revelation when I grasped this concept. I did not want to be skinny anymore so I did research on nutrition and exercise, I applied what I learned and if it did not work I would research some more or ask for help. I did NOT give up, I tried a new approach, experimenting on what worked for me. Slowly I was seeing results, this journey started in 2008 and to this day I'm still learning. I reached my goal, then I made new goals to keep me going. You can achieve your goals as well! You are no exception just a DECISION away from changing your life! Picture yourself standing in front of this mountain, you are trying to reach the top which represents your goals. The problem with most people is they keep staring at how big their mountain is, rationalizing on how difficult and/or impossible to ever get to the top, therefore their mountain seemingly gets bigger. Now they are frozen in fear and do not take any action. Why? What you focus on you magnify. When you focus on the negative, you magnify them resulting in fear and an overbearing feeling of impossibility. What you do instead of staring up at your mountain is look down and take a step and you focus on taking step after step. If you run into an obstacle ask for help then take another step. Focus on the positives along the way, look up every once in a while and celebrate what you achieved so far but continue making steps. Now you are closer to the top, your mountain is shrinking. Don't get too giddy yet stay focused and continue with your steps and when you reach that mountain top you look back and see all the steps you took to get there and how your mountain was not as big as you thought.